Thyroid Diseases

Steps for Improving Your Thyroid Health

TABLE OF CONTENTS

CHAPTER ONE: Thyroid Gland Overview

CHAPTER TWO: Common Thyroid Disorders and Their Causes

CHAPTER THREE: Diagnosis of Thyroid Conditions

CHAPTER FOUR: Treatment and Management of Thyroid Diseases

CHAPTER FIVE: Risk Factors for Thyroid Disorders

CHAPTER SIX: Frequently Asked Questions about Thyroid Health

CHAPTER SEVEN: Conclusion

CHAPTER ONE: Thyroid Gland Overview

The thyroid gland is a 2-inch gland that is located below the Adam's apple (larynx) in the neck region. This organ has two lobes that are connected by the isthmus giving it a bow tie shape. The separate lobes lie on the either sides of the windpipe.

This gland (as a part of the endocrine system) produces thyroid hormones that play a vital role in controlling the body's metabolism, including the energy expenditure within the body and growth. The gland does this by releasing the hormones directly into the bloodstream. In addition, the general endocrine system together with both the nervous and immune systems boosts the body's mechanisms to cope with stress and other external triggers.

Just like the other glands within the body, the pituitary gland (foreseen by the hypothalamus) monitors and regulates the functions of the thyroid gland. Essentially, Iodine is a component for the production of the hormones into the bloodstream. That is, for adequate production of the hormones, the body requires about 150 mcg of iodine each day. Supplementing this iodine is essential for a normal thyroid functioning. The best way to supplement iodine is through the dietary sources of iodine. It is very likely that a healthy body can get rid of an excess iodine when it is consumed from foods.

However, supplementing with iodine as an isolated nutrient can be dangerous because an excess of iodine is as health damaging as being low on it.

Therefore monitoring its intake is advisable by the health practitioners for a healthy thyroid if you decide to take an iodine supplement.

How the thyroid works

THYROID AND PARATHYROID

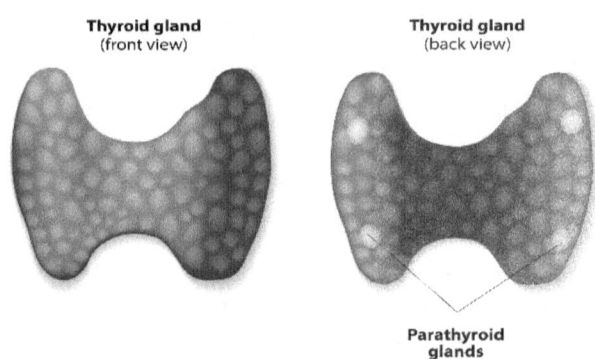

The thyroid is the largest comparing it to the other endocrine glands, and it is the primary regulator of the body's metabolism. This small gland (2 inches) is butterfly-shaped and located at the base of the skull. The physiological functions of this gland are vital in many body processes and developments, including the growth and development in children.

This thyroid works by producing hormones that determine the energy levels as well as the reproduction of every cell. This production of hormones is a complex process that begins from within the brain. Other than managing hunger, sleep, thirst and the body temperature, the hypothalamus regulates the amount of thyroid hormone within the bloodstream.

In the case of low energy levels, the hypothalamus sends the Thyroid Releasing Hormone (TRH) to the pituitary gland, which in turn releases the Thyroid Stimulating Hormone (TSH) that is directed to the thyroid. The thyroid is then triggered to produce the thyroid hormones using the tyrosine amino acid together with iodine. The gland transforms the tyrosine to thyroglobulin that attaches in between one and four iodine atoms to form the T1, T2, T3, and T4 respectively. However, of all the four, the T4 is the storage form of the hormone and hence the primary output of the thyroid before storing them within the tissues for usage when needed.

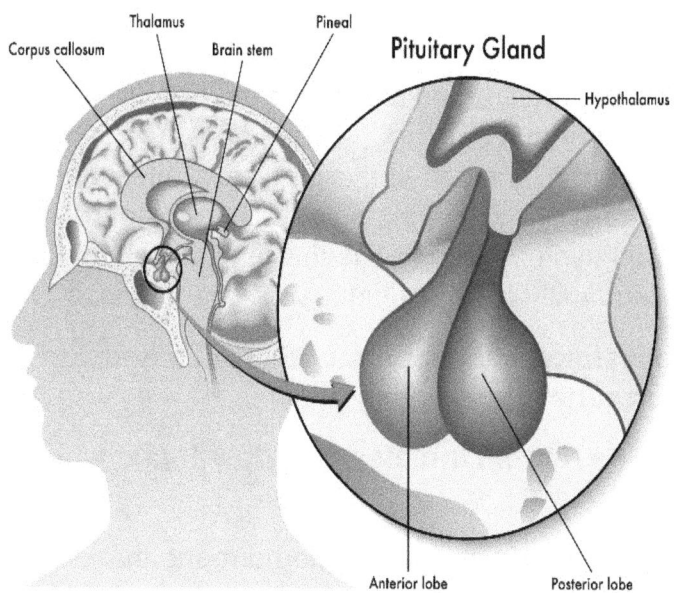

In the case of the low energy level in any part of the body, the T4 is converted to its active form T3 by the help of the deiodinase enzyme. This is done when the deiodinase slices off one iodine atom from the T4 resulting into a free T3 (FT3). The enzyme functions well in the presence of zinc, selenium, and iodine. A portion of the T4 is also used by the by thyroid to form the Reverse T3 (RT3). This results in an inactive form of thyroid that can attach to the receptors of the free T3.

The active T3, with the help of cortisol, enters the cell membrane to control the amount of energy produced by the mitochondria. The T3 acts as the gas pedal to revive power production by the mitochondria while the Reverse T3 acts as the brake pedal to slow down the production of energy in case enough there is more than enough.

All the body's physiological processes require energy for maximum outcome. In the case of a thyroid dysfunction, all the body physiological processes are affected. An array of symptoms that seem not related to thyroid dysfunction. This is the reason why thyroid disease usually goes undiagnosed.

The physiological benefits of thyroid gland and the hormones it produces

1. **The thyroid initiates the growth rate when young**

The thyroid produces the thyroid hormone that other than facilitating metabolism enhances growth. The hormone controls the growth as well as the structure of the bones among the children. At puberty, the hormone helps in sexual development by enhancing a proper conversion of oxygen, sugar, and other body fuels to produce energy.

2. Thyroid acts as the primary center for metabolism

The thyroid is one of the regulators of the body's metabolism. For example, in the presence of enough energy and fat, thyroid hormones enhances the protein anabolism.

3. Thyroid alters the cholesterol levels

It is now clear that the thyroid is essential in metabolic reactions within the body system. Due to this ability, the hormones produced have the ability to break down the harmful cholesterol in order to reduce its concentration within the body tissues.

4. Thyroid enhances the production of energy within the body

Carbohydrates and fat are some of the essential sources of energy within the body. The thyroid ensures that the ingested fat and starch are broken down properly to facilitate the production of energy that would, in turn, facilitate the normal body functioning.

Important facts for improved functioning of the thyroid gland

For one to enjoy the benefits that come along with the thyroid gland, special care has to be taken to enhance its health. Any malfunction of the thyroid gland results in uncontrolled hormone productions and hence thyroid disorders.

Understanding the following tips and relationships is important in maintaining a healthy thyroid for the maximum metabolic processes and hence a healthy living.

Pregnancy and thyroid disorders

The thyroid gland produces hormones that are necessary for normal growth and development of the fetus during pregnancy as well as maintaining the health of the mother. Understanding the effects of pregnancy on the thyroid would be necessary for the pregnant women to protect the health of their fetus.

However, during pregnancy, the thyroid would encounter changes in size and the amount of hormones produced. These changes alter the thyroid glands and its functions.

Fortunately, the thyroid conditions that affect the mothers during pregnancies are normally treatable. The problem comes during the diagnosis of this condition during the pregnancy period because the chief symptoms of the thyroid dysfunction might be the side effects of pregnancy: constipation, fatigue and heat intolerance.

During pregnancy, it is important to take enough iodine to enhance the production of both the maternal and fetal thyroid hormones. This is the reason why most pregnant women are advised to take prenatal vitamins or even better nutrient dense whole foods containing sufficient iodine.

When pregnant, the human chorionic gonadotropin and estrogen cause elevated levels of thyroid hormones within the blood. These hormonal changes make it difficult for a thyroid function tests and interpretations during pregnancy.

Because of this information, research indicates that the women with the thyroid health issues are twice at risk of experiencing miscarriages than those women who do not have the condition. This is helpful in ensuring the health of the pregnant women and the fetus within her.

The Gluten-Thyroid relationship

Studies confirm a positive correlation between the autoimmune thyroid diseases and the gluten intolerance. This means that individuals with autoimmune thyroid conditions like the Hashimoto's are sensitive to gluten. This is because of the similarity in molecular structure between the gliadin (protein portion of gluten) and the transglutaminase (the enzyme responsible for the formation of chemical bonds throughout the whole body) found in the thyroid.

Upon the ingestion of the gliadin, it is absorbed into the bloodstream producing the antibodies against the foreign agent. Because of the molecular similarity to the transglutaminase, however, the antibodies end up attacking the thyroid for up to 6 months after the gluten consumption.

Because of the disturbed thyroid physiology, the general health of the body is altered thereby resulting in poor hormone synthesis and metabolism. This is the reason why nutritional interventions (like cutting the gluten from the normal diet) are important for individuals with chronic autoimmune disorders.

Being that thyroid malfunction contributes to the general body ill-health, it is important to consider some six facts to confirm whether gluten is the main cause of the autoimmune issue:

> ### Gut health tests

Specific stool and blood lab tests are vital to determine the health of the microbiome within the gut. This is important in ruling out the leaky gut or intestinal permeability. Stool analysis is preferred to blood analysis because the condition is detected early before it is absorbed into the bloodstream.

Upon identifying gluten sensitivity in an individual, it is important to apply specific nutritional interventions early enough to curb the adverse conditions.

> ### Comprehensive gluten intolerance labs

It is reported that to determine gluten sensitivity is not easy due to many reasons. For example, most health practitioners conduct only the alpha gliadin tests that usually indicate that there is no issue with the thyroid health.

Knowing this, studies advise that a comprehensive test is conducted to produce accurate insight of a condition. This would also allow us to determine whether the thyroid malfunction is the main cause or not.

> **Avoiding other triggers for autoimmune thyroid issues**

Research shows that autoimmune issues might result from a combination of both the genetic vulnerability and environmental triggers. Therefore, understanding the different causes of autoimmune issues is the first step involved in the protection of the general health. Other than gluten, the other identified triggers of autoimmune conditions include infection, stress, artificial sweeteners, iodine and smoking among other unlimited contributing factors.

Relationship between stress and thyroid autoimmunity

The thyroid requires a regulated amount of stress hormones to function normally. However, studies indicate that both the physiological and psychological stressors induce the various immunological alterations. That is, stress might result in either the overproduction or underproduction of hormones and hence a negative effect on the thyroid gland.

In the case of any kind of stress, the brain releases the corticotropin-releasing hormones (CRH) that trigger the pituitary to produce the TSH, which in turn influences the adrenal glands to release cortisol. Both the CRH and the cortisol might inhibit the production of TSH as well as the conversion of T4 to T3. This might lead to symptoms like weight gain, fatigue, poor concentration, infertility among other conditions.

With this in mind, it is good to avoid any kind of stress that would eventually result in an adrenal imbalance. Resetting your stress response reestablishes the communication along the brain-adrenal-thyroid pathway.

CHAPTER TWO: Common Thyroid Disorders and Their Causes

The American Thyroid Association indicates that about 20 million Americans suffer from thyroid diseases with 60% unaware of their conditions because of the difficulty involved in determining the root causes. This is evident by the increasing incidences and prevalence of these chronic diseases in the United States.

Thyroid conditions occur because of either the underactive or the overactive thyroid glands: hypothyroidism or hyperthyroidism respectively. For instance, research indicates that a higher percentage of the thyroid conditions result due to poisoning by fluoride present in water. Just like chlorine, fluorine impedes the iodine receptors within the thyroid glands resulting in reduced hormone production and hence hypothyroidism. Other than the fluoride, stimulants such as tea, coffee, and alcohol also have the ability to cause imbalances because it disrupts your glandular system.

Genetic factors, pregnancy, stress, nutritional imbalances, environmental toxins and autoimmune attacks are some of the outlined causes responsible for the thyroid functioning going haywire. These thyroid disorders can range from the small' harmless goiter to life-threatening cancer.

Hypothyroidism

This one class of the thyroid conditions occurs when the thyroid produces less amount of thyroid hormones

into the blood stream. The less hormone production is due to the underactive thyroid glands.
Underproduction of thyroid hormones would mean that less energy is produced to facilitate the cellular activities within the entire body.

Any problem within either your pituitary gland, hypothalamus or the thyroid gland can result in the little production of the thyroid hormones. To help in the appropriate diagnosis, there are certain symptoms that indicate this hormonal imbalance: fatigue, poor concentration, feeling cold, constipation, fluid retention, ache in the joints and muscles, depression, irregular menstruation, weight gain as well as a dry hair and skin.

There are different causes that might result to this underproduction of the thyroid hormones into the bloodstream. This abnormal underproduction leads to imbalanced chemical reactions within the body. Examples include the autoimmune diseases, radiotherapy, thyroid surgery, treatment of the hyperthyroidism among other thyroid medications.

1. Autoimmune diseases

In the case of an abnormal body physiological functioning, the immune system might produce antibodies against the body's own tissues. With increasing scientific support, scientists argue that bacteria and virus might be the reasons for the ill-functioning of the immune system. Other than the many other triggers for such a response, genetic history also plays a role.

During this response, the immune system might also produce antibodies against the thyroid gland and hence resulting to the reduced production of the metabolic hormones. For example, the Hashimoto's thyroiditis, that occurs when the immune system attacks the thyroid glands, is a common cause of the hypothyroidism. This condition, characterized by thyroid inflammation, is chronic and remains stable for up to 5 years before its signs manifest. This Hashimoto disease is common in people with histories of other immune conditions like the type 1 diabetes or the vitiligo.

2. Medications' side effects

In the case of hyperthyroidism, the health practitioners recommend medication aimed at reducing the amount of thyroid hormones within the bloodstream. Some of these interventions result in complications that predispose an individual to hypothyroidism.

For example, the anti-thyroid medication aimed at managing hyperthyroidism or even the thyroid cancer might alter the functioning of the gland and hence reducing the amount of hormone it produces into the bloodstream.

In addition to the anti-thyroid medication, the radioactive iodine is used to destruct the thyroid to manage both the hyperthyroidism and the thyroid cancer.

The intake of these hyperthyroidism medications, therefore, must be monitored since, in excess, they might result in a permanent hypothyroidism. Because of this, it is advisable to consult professional health practitioners to recommend and help you monitor the usage of the reliable quality medication against hyperthyroidism.

3. Congenital diseases

Due to some unknown reasons, some babies are born with defective body organs. However, some of them inherit the conditions from their parents.

In connection to thyroid disorders, however, some children are born with dysfunctional thyroids or sometimes with no thyroid glands at all. This results in less production of thyroid hormones for metabolic functions. These children deal with the delayed development of permanent teeth, poor mental development, poor growth as well as the delayed onset of puberty.

To show how this condition is serious, research indicates that up to 1 in 3,000 babies suffer from this uncommon congenital hypothyroidism.

4. Thyroid surgery

One intervention against thyroid disorders is the removal of the thyroid. However, the surgical removal of a relatively large portion of the thyroid gland alters the hormone production of the gland and hence less concentration within the body cells for maximum metabolism.

To substitute this and ensure you live a life free of hypothyroidism, physicians recommend thyroid hormones supplements for the remaining part of your life.

5. Abnormal growths in the thyroid

Due to factors like the autoimmune disorders, abnormal growths might invade the thyroid and as a result, replace the healthy tissue. These growths hinder the production of enough thyroid hormones for metabolism. This is hypothyroidism.

The best way to control this is to curb the risk factors such as the autoimmune diseases to protect the thyroid.

The abnormal growth can, therefore, be removed surgically to reverse the adverse effects that might be experienced.

6. Problem in the pituitary

Other than the actual thyroid gland, hypothyroidism might occur because of problems with the pituitary glands. For example, the thyroid gland might produce fewer hormones because of lack of communication from the pituitary glands. This can be because of failure of the pituitary gland to produce the Thyroid Stimulating Hormones (TSH) that trigger the production of the T4 by the thyroid gland.

7. Genetic defects

Considering the genetic makeup of an individual, some children are born with congenital hypothyroidism. This can be because of lack of a regulatory gene to facilitate the production of the thyroid hormones.

For the management, it is recommendable to diagnose the children with this condition early enough to recommend the use of thyroid hormone supplements for a happy living.

To manage this hypothyroidism condition. Therefore, the patients diagnosed with the underproduction of thyroid hormones are advised to take hormone tablets each day to replace the hormones that the thyroid is not making.

Hyperthyroidism

Just as the name suggests, this class of thyroid dysfunction entails the thyroid overproducing the thyroid hormones that regulate how our body cells utilize the energy. When our thyroid is overactive, the body's processes speed up, and you may experience anxiety, hand tremor, weight loss, rapid heartbeat, difficulty in sleeping and body weakness among other adverse symptoms.

Many underlying factors are responsible for the excess production of the thyroid hormones and hence excessively high metabolic rate. Knowing the causes of this condition is necessary for its reliable management.

1. Autoimmune diseases

Autoimmune conditions result when the immune system produces antibodies against the healthy tissues of the thyroid gland. This can result in either an underactive or an overactive thyroid-altering the metabolic processes as a result.

Graves' disease is an example of the autoimmune disorders that interferes with the thyroid gland to produce excess hormones for metabolism. This condition occurs when the immune system produces the Thyroid-stimulating immunoglobulins (TSIs) antibodies that attack the thyroid by binding to its receptors. This replacement of the TSH by the TSIs tricks the thyroid to produce too many hormones into the bloodstream. This disease might result in an enlarged thyroid gland (thyrotoxic goiter), skin thickening and eye problem. Diagnosing this condition is difficult hence the need to take heed of the symptoms for early interventions. Other autoimmune conditions responsible for this hyperthyroidism include the Plummer's disease and the thyroiditis.

2. Hyperfunctioning thyroid nodules

Adenomas, a part of the thyroid gland that walls itself from the rest of the gland, forms a benign tumor that results in the enlargement of the thyroid. These toxic adenomas might produce many hormones than required by the body and hence an imbalanced metabolic rate. This condition is what is referred to as Plummer's disease.

Not all adenomas produce excess hormones. However, no research has been able to explain the exact causes that trigger them to produce the excess thyroid hormones.

3. Thyroiditis

Because of an infection or due to the problems with the immune system, the thyroid gland can become inflamed causing excess thyroid hormones stored within the gland to leak into the bloodstream. This results in increased metabolic processes and hence the body processes.

There are many types of this thyroiditis conditions. Other than the rare granulomatous thyroiditis and the subacute thyroiditis, the other thyroiditis is harmless and mostly occurs after pregnancy in women (postpartum thyroiditis).

4. Excess iodine

Iodine is an essential element required by the thyroid to manufacture the thyroid hormones for enhanced metabolism. The gland cannot produce its own iodine hence the need to add it as a supplement into the body in the correct amount.

This iodine supplementation is an intervention used to manage hypothyroidism. That is, the drugs such as the amiodarone given as medication against irregular heartbeats are some of the medications with high iodine concentration.

However, the use of these medications should be controlled. This is because recent research indicates that consuming substances high in iodine concentration prove to be disastrous to the useful thyroid health. To curb these adverse effects, it is advisable to take keen consideration the prescriptions by a qualified physician.

Complications resulting from unmanaged hyperthyroidism

The elevated rate of metabolism affects the speed of the general body processes. This might result in several complications among the affected.

- ✓ **Brittle bones**

Calcium and other minerals when incorporated into the bones enhance the strength of the skeletal framework. The absorption of these minerals into the bones is facilitated by the thyroid hormones produced by the thyroid glands.

Too much of thyroid hormones, therefore, interferes with the body's ability to utilize the minerals for strong bones. This results in weak and brittle bones (osteoporosis).

✓ Loss of vision

Individuals with Graves' disease, a condition associated with hyperthyroidism, develop eye problems, including sensitivity to light, swollen eyes and blurred vision among several others. If not treated early enough, severe eye conditions might lead to a permanent loss of vision.

✓ Heart problems

Hyperthyroidism results in increased rates of the body's metabolic processes. This is evidenced by the rapid heart rates as well as a heart rhythm disorder (atrial fibrillation). In addition to these heart conditions, the heart fails to circulate enough blood within the body.

Fortunately, the associated heart problems are reversible if special treatments are taken into consideration.

✓ Thyrotoxic crisis

In case the health problems associated thyroid condition, hyperthyroidism suddenly intensifies the symptoms if not managed early enough. This is a thyrotoxic crisis. This would as a result lead to fever, delirium as well as a rapid pulse rate.

This sudden onset requires that you seek immediate medical attention from the qualified health practitioners.

- ✓ **Skin conditions**

Autoimmune disorders such as the Graves' disease have adverse effects on the skin if not controlled early enough. For instance, the Graves' dermopathy, common in individuals with Graves' disease, causes the skin to swell and turn red, particularly on the feet and shins.

CHAPTER THREE: Diagnosis of Thyroid Conditions

Symptoms of the various thyroid conditions are non-specific making it difficult to diagnose them. This is the reason for the increased incidences and prevalence of this chronic condition in the United States according to reports by the American Thyroid Association (ATA). Because of this, the primary health practitioners advocate for early diagnosis and treatment of these disorders to ascertain the root cause of the unusual symptoms.

The health professionals focus on the cardiac, skin, vision and neurologic findings to determine any problem with the thyroid gland. Different tests and scans are conducted depending on the initial results.

Doctors measure the levels of hormones (both the thyroid hormones and the Thyroid Stimulating) within the bloodstream in order to diagnose any thyroid condition. The first test entails the determination of the amount of thyroid stimulating hormones within the blood. That is, an excessive amount of TSH in the blood indicates that the metabolic malfunctions are due to overproduction of these hormones while lower readings (below the normal amounts) indicates that the gland is not producing enough amounts of theses hormones. Other blood tests such as the Free T4, Antithyroid antibody, as well as the TSH receptor antibody tests can also be done to ascertain the hormone concentrations in the bloodstream.

In addition to the blood tests, a nuclear thyroid scan can be done by swallowing regulated radioactive iodine. Any decrease or increase in iodine update indicates a hypothyroidism and hyperthyroidism respectively. For this scan, the radioactive iodine can as well be introduced into the body through injection.

Another way to determine any malfunction in the thyroid glands is the presence of nodules present within the gland. This is done by conducting a thyroid ultrasound examination of the gland. This painless procedure utilizes the sound waves in order to generate the images of the thyroid to help determine any thyroid abnormalities (presence of cysts, tumors, and nodules). As a result, this intervention can also examine either an underactive or overactive thyroid glands. As an advantage, health practitioners use this thyroid ultrasound as an overall physical examination. This is because the hormones produced by the thyroid glands regulate all the metabolic conditions hence the general health.

Another testing procedure entails the doctor obtaining a sample from the thyroid using a fine-needle aspiration. This is done under the guidance of ultrasound test. The sample obtained is examined under a microscope with high resolving power to help determine any condition of the thyroid such as the thyroid cancer.

Thyroid disease and family history. Studies indicate that thyroid disorders are genetic. It is, therefore, important to give every information about your personal medical history as well as the family history concerning thyroid health. Qualified and experienced health providers might use your history to determine whether you are suffering from the thyroid diseases.

Physical examination of the thyroid gland is another way of determining your thyroid health. This involves a thorough examination by observing the physical symptoms of a malfunctioning thyroid.

A systematic approach before booking an appointment for thyroid diagnosis

Misdiagnosis of thyroid conditions has adverse effects on the general body health just like explained in the earlier chapter of this book. It is, therefore, important not to miss a diagnosis of hyperthyroidism or hypothyroidism. To ascertain this, professional physicians advise the public to consider a systematic and proven appointment procedure to ensure you get valid diagnosis results for a healthy thyroid.

- Before deciding to book an appointment with your health practitioner, the first step involves going through your previous thyroid test. In the United Kingdom, for example, you have the right to access your medical records under the Data Protection Act of 1998.
- Insist on actual figures of your thyroid test results. Do not accept the 'normal' answer. This is because the test ranges differ in the different geographical jurisdiction. That is, a range in one country might be 0.4 - 4.0 while in another country 0.5 - 5.0. For example, a test result above or below 10 might be a good idea to share with your personal doctor to give him or her a clue on what diagnosis procedures to consider.
- Ensure the thyroid test is conducted at the same time of the day every time you are

testing for the thyroid hormone levels. This is because of the circadian rhythm whose levels differ at different times of the day. For example, the TSH level is at peak between midnight and 6 am.
- Embrace the need to have a diary to help you indicate your health progress. The diary should include, therefore, the thyroid test dates, results, and their ranges. A positive trend motivates you to ensure a healthy thyroid as well as gives the doctors the go ahead to select the intervention options that fits for your healthy thyroid and the general body health.
- Self-analyze yourself to identify the symptoms of a thyroid disorder (either hypothyroidism or the hyperthyroidism) then tick them off on a Thyroid Disorder Symptom List provided by your health provider. Rate the symptoms in the range 1- 10 with 10 being the worst. This is done at regular intervals (at the same time the tests are done).
- Read the various publications about the thyroid health to be informed on these conditions. Highlight the relevant areas to show your physician.
- Prepare a list of questions to ask your doctor considering your thyroid health. This would help you further understand your personal thyroid health.

Reasons for frequent misdiagnosis of thyroid disorders

With the estimation by the Thyroid Federation International that about half the global population with thyroid conditions are unaware of their suffering. Many people with this chronic condition are left suffering from the accompanying life-threatening symptoms due to misdiagnosis of these thyroid conditions.

This information called for the researchers to conduct studies on the various reasons for the frequent misdiagnosis of these chronic disorders.

i. Incompetent health professional

Trained health practitioners understand the need to conduct a comprehensive blood testing before considering the various interventions for the management of the undesirable thyroid conditions. Incompetent doctors were found to rely on the FSH and the T4 test result alone. With this, they end up assuming that our bodies convert all the T4 to the active T3.

ii. Outdated TSH test ranges

Many traditional thyroid doctors operate with the reading of between 0.5 – 5.0 regardless of the patients' obvious symptoms. Most recent studies indicate that the range varies from different laboratories in different countries globally.

However, the modern integrative thyroid advocate strives to fight for a narrow lab range. All health professionals should also endeavor to maintain a narrower range in their fight against thyroid conditions.

iii. Failure to recognize the warning symptoms of thyroid disorders

The thyroid gland is the ultimate engine for the general body metabolism. This means that any thyroid malfunction would result to general body flopping. Because of the obvious symptoms such as the fatigue, swollen eyes as well as slowed reflexes, most sufferers, and the health practitioners fail to notice the presence of thyroid conditions.

Professional physicians also found out that the body temperature is a more reliable determinant of thyroid disorders compared to the standard test ranges. However, the body's sensitivity and accuracy to the thermometer required for the temperature reading makes it not possible to acquire reliable outcomes.

It is, therefore, the responsibility of both you and the health providers to determine the thyroid health for special interventions to be taken into consideration.

CHAPTER FOUR: Treatment and Management of Thyroid Diseases

The thyroid gland produces hormones that facilitate every metabolic process within the body. The energy produced drives all the body functions for healthy living. Any malfunction of the thyroid gland would result to altered body physiological process. Of the many thyroid conditions, hyperthyroidism (because of an overactive thyroid) and hypothyroidism (results from an underactive thyroid) are the most common.

Fortunately, many thyroid remedies in the market make use of both the natural and the supplementations to maintain the thyroid health. It is, however, important to determine first the type and causes of the thyroid disorder you are suffering from before opting to treat it. For example, the autoimmune thyroid disorder occurs when the immune system mistakenly attacks the thyroid gland. This assumption of the actual cause of the conditions such as the autoimmune disorders would only result in a continuous loss more thyroid cell thereby increasing the requirements for the thyroid replacement hormones.

After a successful diagnosis, evaluation of the specific lab tests is done to develop a Neuro-Metabolic Treatment (NMT) plan that is all-inclusive and with four key elements:

- ❖ **Modified lifestyle**

For proper functioning of the thyroid gland in the synthesis of energy for the general body physiological process, regulated amount of stress hormones is also required. Adrenal glands balance the blood sugar level when the body is under stress. Too much of the stress hormones, however, result in an imbalanced thyroid functioning and hence altered body processes.

Changing your lifestyle is an ideal measure to reduce stress on the various body systems and glands. This would mean as a result enhances the healing process by the adrenal gland since the blood sugar levels are maintained.

- ❖ **Modified dieting**

Some foods taken into the body might contribute to the experienced thyroid conditions affecting the globe. That is, the foods and herbs cause an imbalance of the immune system. The immune system would in the process attack the thyroid cells causing the various autoimmune disorders like the Graves' disease.

Once an adverse condition is identified during the diagnosis, the health practitioners have to advise their clients on the specific foods (for example foods rich in protein) that help the immune system regain its balance for a healthy thyroid and body in general.

- ❖ **Use of nutritional supplements**

In addition to both the lifestyle and diet modifications, adding the various nutritional supplements would ensure a fast and smooth healing and recovery process. These add-ons do this by cutting short the time required for the immune system to regain its balance.

The professionals explain the importance of supplements in hastening the recovery process. They, as a result, provide the victims of the various thyroid conditions with the recommended supplements for a healthy thyroid gland.

- ❖ **Brain Based Therapy**

A modified and carefully monitored Brain Based Therapy protocol is necessary for the purpose to reset the thyroid gland for a healthy body. This is usually based on a functional neurological examination.

Critically following the four-step approach provides a foundation through which the body regains its balance.

However, the Neuro-Metabolic Treatment (NMT) plan depends largely on a specific type of thyroid malfunction realized during the diagnosis. That is, when treating hyperthyroidism, the manufacture of the thyroid hormones is suppressed while for hypothyroidism, hormone replacement is the ultimate goal of the health practitioners. Before deciding on the effective treatment strategy, conventional medicines offer effective techniques for eliminating, supplementing as well as lowering hormone production by the thyroid gland.

Based on your specific thyroid outcome, the doctor recommends the intervention strategies that would ensure a balanced thyroid gland.

Treatment options for hyperthyroidism

Hyperthyroidism occurs in the case of an overactive thyroid that results in the production of more than enough thyroid hormones into the bloodstream. In this scenario, the health practitioners strive to suppress the hormone synthesis by the gland. The doctors understand the reliable strategies that would be of help in this area: anti-thyroid medication, radioiodine treatment, and surgery.

- **The use of radioiodine as a treatment for hyperthyroidism**

This is a form of radiotherapy involving the ingestion of tablet or liquid medication containing radioactive iodine. The radioactive element damages the thyroid cells in order to limit or destroy their ability to produce hormones.

However, due to the proven effects of radioactive substances on the body tissues, it is advisable for the women to avoid conceiving for a minimum of six months after treatment and the men should not father a child for about four months after the treatment. This method of treating hyperthyroidism is not recommended for both the breastfeeding and pregnant mothers.

Once you are treated using this strategy, regular thyroid checkups are necessary since many people eventually experience the effects of an underactive thyroid. This is because of the principle destruction of the thyroid cells by when this treatment option is considered.

To curb the adverse effects that come along with the use of radioiodine, the other medical interventions against this overproduction of hormones are occasionally needed to effectively restore the normal hormone synthesis by the thyroid into the bloodstream.

The use of anti-thyroid medications

There are many medications against the thyroid. Just as the name suggests, anti-thyroid medications (carbimazole or propylthiouracil) interfere with the normal functions of the thyroid to produce hormones. Upon considering this type of treatment option, the hyperthyroidism symptoms disappears after about four weeks after the dose starts to impair the production of hormones by the thyroid gland.

There are two different procedures for using this medication. The first one involves giving very high doses of the anti-thyroid medications to stop further production of hormones. Thyroid tablets are then used to supplement the hormones. The second treatment option involves giving a controlled amount of anti-thyroid medication while regularly monitoring the outcome until a normal hormone level is achieved. Immediately the thyroid function is restored, the dosage of this medication is gradually reduced to minimize any chances of side effects.

A rare but serious side effect observed in those under this type of medication is agranulocytosis, which involves the reduced production of white cells by the bone marrow. The one symptom of this condition is a sore throat. This, therefore, means that in case you experience a sore throat when under this medication, visit your personal doctor to confirm whether your white cells are good.

Surgical removal of the thyroid gland

Surgery of the thyroid is advisable when the cause of the hyperthyroidism is the toxic adenomas. This is because the adenomas nodules are resistant to the radioiodine medication. These nodules are common in persons below the age of 45 years old. This permanent medication is also necessary in the case where the other medications have failed to balance the thyroid health.

After the malfunctioning thyroid tissue is surgically removed, the hormone level normal in few weeks. Monitoring must be done during this time as many patients become hypothyroid over time. Other side effects of surgery include neck swelling at the point of incision, difficulty in swallowing, discomfort at the back of the neck among other undesirable effects.

The Treatment Options for Hypothyroidism

This thyroid condition occurs when the thyroid produces less amount of hormones into the bloodstream hence slowed body physiological processes. Managing this condition thereby involves any strategy that is aimed at supplementing the fewer hormones (thyroid hormone replacement). Unlike in hyperthyroidism, conventional treatment measures cannot boost the thyroid gland to produce more hormones for metabolism.

Although there are many hormones from animal extract, professional physicians prefer the synthetic forms of thyroid hormone. However, one can choose from many treatment options available. The three common strategies communally applied include the use of synthetic thyroid hormone, the natural thyroid hormones, and the natural treatment methods.

The use of synthetic Thyroid Hormone

Most physicians recommend this common thyroid intervention for their clients with low production of the thyroid hormones. An example of these synthetic thyroid hormones includes the levothyroxine and Synthroid among the many other available brands of this medication. These synthetic hormones are made of both the thyroxin (T3) and the triiodothyronine (T4). Victims take the hormone therapy with either drugs or the injection.

The synthetic thyroid hormones have been proven to effectively manage the symptoms of thyroid malfunction with minimal side effects. However, adjusting the dose of medication alleviates any undesirable effects that come along with these synthetic medication products.

Using this treatment option does not alleviate the root cause of the low production of thyroid hormones by the thyroid. For instance, not all thyroid condition are because of thyroid gland malfunction. The synthetic thyroid hormone would help in managing the symptoms but not the underlying cause of the problem.

The use of Natural Thyroid Hormones

Like mentioned earlier, there are hormones that come from either the animal and plant extract. Examples of such medical remedy hormones include the Westhroid and the Armour. Many holistic doctors recommend the natural thyroid hormones. This is because it has minimal side effects compared to the synthetic thyroid hormones.

For those individuals who do not do well with the synthetic thyroid hormones, the natural thyroid hormones are known to be the best option. This type of hypothyroidism management procedure is preferred to the synthetic option since many see it as 'natural' despite the fact that it cannot be similar to the ones our bodies produce. The hormone remedy works well within our glands compared to the 'synthetic' hormones

Just like the synthetic thyroid hormone, however, the natural thyroid hormone does not alleviate the underlying causes of the thyroid conditions.

The use of the Natural Treatment Methods

The thyroid treatment options discussed above have no ability to relieve the root cause of the experienced hypothyroidism. The goal of this treatment method, however, is to restore a person's health back to normal. This is the reason why most people globally prefer this method as the ultimate solution to manage their hypothyroidism.

Under proper supervision by a qualified physician, the natural treatment methods have resulted in a recommendable outcome that appeals to many. It has shown to have greater health benefits of all the hypothyroidism management strategies.

The only negative thing with these types of treatments is taking responsibility for your own health, unlike the other two methods that only involves taking pills or injections.

In general, selecting the best treatment method for your underactive thyroid depends on your own preference. However, try all the available medical intervention and then choose the one that gives you the outcome you desire.

CHAPTER FIVE: Risk Factors for Thyroid Disorders

The various thyroid conditions are because of an imbalance of the hormones within the body. This can result because the thyroid produces either too much (hyperthyroidism) or too little thyroid hormones (hypothyroidism).

These thyroid conditions are not preventable making them hard to manage diseases. However, having awareness about the potential risk factors helps your doctor establish the need for screening to prevent the complications that might come along with these health issues.

Many factors expose the general population to these diseases with undesirable symptoms and complications.

A. Age

Thyroid disorders have no age limits. At any age, one is at a risk of getting these thyroid conditions. However, research indicates that the disorders are common among the elderly (50 years and above). To minimize the complications that come along with the dysfunctional thyroid gland, older patients require special care and regular follow-up. As support for this, research shows that most thyroid patients are elderly.

B. Gender

To start with, Edward Toromanyan (a member of the Armenian Ministry of Health) recorded that women are 3 times at risk of experiencing this health problem than men. This was attributed to the susceptibility of women to hormonal fluctuations. That is, iodine deficiency causes adverse complications to the female, and not in males. Pregnant women experience serious hormonal changes and hence more sensitive to iodine sensitivity.

Health professionals advise the women on the importance of embracing the consumption of the iodized salt as well as regular ultrasound screening of the thyroid for an early detection of any thyroid condition.

C. Family history

Research shows that existence of an individual with thyroid condition increases the chances of the others in the same lineage to suffer from a similar thyroid disease. The risk is believed to be greater if there is a first-degree female relative with a thyroid condition. This, therefore, means that it is important to be aware of your family history of the thyroid conditions.

D. Cigarette smoking

Our own choices might increase our chances of facing the complications of the thyroid illnesses. Cigarette smoking, for example, is a drive for the thyroid disorders since tobacco contains thiocyanate chemical that acts as an anti-thyroid agent. This tobacco smoking worsens the complications of the various autoimmune conditions such as Graves' diseases and hence reducing the effectiveness of treatment for thyroid eye disease.

E. Treatment of hyperthyroidism or Graves' disease

There are many strategies used to manage the complications of hyperthyroidism. For example, surgical removal of a part or the whole thyroid is an intervention to prevent hyperthyroidism. Radioactive Iodine Treatment used to treat the Graves' disease as well as the thyroid cancer leads to the destruction of the thyroid cells hence increasing the chances of facing hypothyroidism.

But before thinking about the above treatments you owe it to yourself and see first if Autoimmunity might be the primary suspicious here. If you have autoimmunity where the immune system is creating antibodies to attack the thyroid gland, this might lead to hyperthyroidism. One of the antibodies that cause Graves' disease is thyroid-stimulating immunoglobulins (1). So you need to find out if you have some type of autoimmune disease which probably being caused by intestinal permeability (also known as Leaky Gut).

F. Neck surgery

Neck surgery, biopsy or even injection in the neck region might cause trauma to the thyroid gland. This increases the chances of an individual to suffer from the adverse health effects of a dysfunctional thyroid.

Exposure to surgical antiseptic such as iodine can also increase your chances of temporary thyroid malfunction (either hyperthyroidism or hypothyroidism). The individuals with underlying thyroid antibodies are at a greater risk of suffering from the thyroid health conditions.

G. Consumption of goitrogenic foods

Many plant foods contain goitrogen chemicals that are known to promote the enlargement of the thyroid (goiter). Examples of such foods include cabbage, turnips, okra, cilantro, kohlrabi and Brussels sprout among several others.

This phytochemical negatively affect the absorption of iodine which is a crucial mineral the thyroid gland needs to function normally. And this is especially damaging for individuals who consume a low amount of iodine in their diets in the first place. It is recommended to eat small amounts of these types of vegetables and even better to increase your uptake of iodine through the consumption of seaweed that is rich in iodine. Cooking such as boiling vegetables and discarding the water will minimize the number of goitrogens in them significantly. Also, fermenting vegetables can reduce the amount of certain goitrogens such as nitrils but probably not as effective as a cooking method, so you need to be careful consuming too much fermented cruciferous vegetables.

H. Stress

For proper functioning of the thyroid gland, some regulated amount of stress hormones is required. This makes the adrenal gland an important organ for the general body functions.

However, major stress – either emotional or physical might trigger the thyroid gland to malfunction. That is, either produce little (hypothyroidism) or excess hormones (hyperthyroidism).

I. Iodine intake

Iodine is an important element in the production of thyroid hormones for body metabolic functions. However, too much or deficient iodine prove to be disastrous to the thyroid. To maintain a healthy thyroid. Therefore, it is important to regulate your iodine intake. Many scientist and functional doctors recommend supplementing iodine from whole foods such as seaweed and certain types of fish (particularly fish heads) that are naturally rich in iodine. It seems the body can get rid of any excess iodine when it is consumed that way rather taking an isolated iodine supplement, especially for the long term.

J. Exposure to radiation

For the treatment of both the head and neck cancer, medical practitioners expose the head and neck respectively to radiation. This might cause thyroid trauma hence malfunctioning.

Other than the medical radiation, people accidently are exposed to the environmental radiation. For example, accidental ingesting the radiation-contaminated foods. The radiations increase the chances of autoimmune conditions.

K. Personal history of the thyroid condition

Studies indicate that the individuals with a history of autoimmune diseases are at a greater risk of experiencing the complications of the malfunctioning thyroid once again. With this in mind, it is important to take precaution in case you have such a history.

Like earlier, stated, knowing your level of risk for thyroid disease and informing your physician is an indication that you are in the right direction towards a healthy thyroid. This also allows for early diagnosis and detection and hence early treatment before the complications worsen.

CHAPTER SIX: Questions and Answers

In this chapter, I am going to answer some frequent (and some not so frequent but important) questions about thyroid gland health and disorders.

Q1: What some of the foods are rich in iodine?

A1: sea vegetables are rich in iodine, but they vary from one type to another. The method of drying seaweeds can affect the content of iodine since sun-dried seaweeds can vaporize a significant amount iodine. Seaweeds such as Hijiki, Kelp, knotten wrack, Wakame, Arame, and Kombu.

Asparagus, garlic, leafy greens like spinach, Lima and navy beans, mushrooms, pineapple, and strawberries. Coconuts because they grow close to the ocean are considered to be a decent source of iodine too.

Dairy products such as butter and yogurt can provide a good amount of iodine if these cows are eating their natural food of different types of grass which is grown in soil rich in iodine.

Sea fish like whiting, cod, haddock and sardines. Shellfish, like oysters, clams, lobster, and mussels.

Q2: How do I know if I am deficient in iodine?

A2: One way is to use an iodine skin tincture such as Lugol.

Apply a patch iodine solution (about the size of your palm) on your skin, that way you'll have a brown pigment on your skin. If the iodine pigment on your skin gets absorbed thus, disappear then that most likely explains you have a certain level of iodine deficiency.

Q3: How Does an intestinal permeability can cause thyroid disorders such as hypothyroidism or hyperthyroidism?

A3: In general, having some degree of leaky gut (or intestinal permeability) which means incomplete digested foods and microorganism toxins can leak through the gut to the bloodstream. When immune cells encounter these partially digested foods and toxins will start to attack them and create antibodies. When toxins, for example, get attached to the tissues such as the thyroid gland, then the immune system will attack the thyroid gland tissue causing hypothyroidism and to a lesser degree hyperthyroidism.

Q4: Can someone have normal production of thyroid hormones but still have a thyroid disorder?

A4: There are cases when the thyroid hormone production is normal however due to toxins that likely caused by leaky gut syndrome. These toxins are binding to thyroid hormone receptors. Therefore, the hormones cannot enter the cells and fulfill their purpose. And patients can be misdiagnosed as having hypothyroidism (2 - page 144).

Q5: When iodine supplement and hormone replacements are considered not a good solution?

A5: In the past, many countries around the world had (and some still do) deficiency in trace mineral iodine and all sort of iodine-deficiency health disorders became prevalent in these countries. Some of the solutions were to use iodized salt and including iodine in drinking water. Which worked great for the most part, however, many patients with thyroid disorders have an autoimmune disease and not necessarily lack of iodine intake.

The ingesting excessive amount of iodine can trigger an autoimmune disorder and the second issue is that you probably don't have iodine deficiency but have an autoimmune disorder caused by the digestive disorder. That is why it is critical to have the correct diagnosis so you can treat your thyroid disorder effectively and as safely as possible.

Q6: How to maintain a healthy thyroid gland?

A6: That's the one-million dollar question! From researching on this subject for many years now, it is essential to understand the environmental toxins we are exposed to and foods that we eat are major factors, however, are not the only factors damaging the thyroid gland and other body organs for that matter. Here are few points you need to consider:

1-Avoid Bromide chemical with many types of forms. Bromide can bind to the same receptors that are used in the thyroid gland to absorb iodine. Potassium Bromate is a dough conditioner used in baked goods that are sold in the U.S. and other countries.

Methyl Bromide is a type of pesticide used in agriculture and conventional strawberries (and possibly organic strawberries too) and sprayed with this chemical.

2-Make sure you eat foods that have a decent amount of iodine.

3- Chlorine and fluoride are toxic chemicals and can compete with iodine receptors in the thyroid gland so filtering your drinking and shower water is a wise step toward a healthy thyroid gland.

4-Besides the trace mineral iodine, foods that rich in selenium are important since Selenium is also essential for the conversion of T4 to T3 which is the active form of thyroid hormone. Vitamin A and zinc and magnesium minerals are also found to play a critical role in the thyroid hormone production.

5- Make sure you have a healthy digestive system to prevent a leaky gut where science is discovering how the gut has a significant on the thyroid gland and many other organs in the body. It is amazing more than two thousand years ago that shows how Hippocrates was correct when he said: "All diseases begin in the gut."

6- Overburdened adrenal glands can have an indirect negative effect on your thyroid gland by affecting the pituitary gland through a physiological mechanism called hypothalamic-pituitary-adrenal (HPA) axis and very likely other tissues in the body.

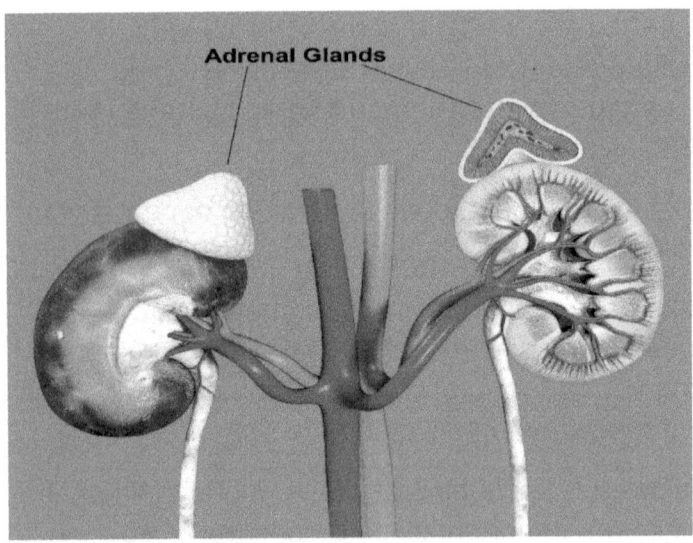

Therefore, in some cases the health of the thyroid gland is normal but having adrenal gland problems affecting the pituitary gland leading to thyroid dysfunction (3).

One of the major roles of the pituitary gland is when detecting there is little thyroid hormone secretion is to produce a **thyrotropin** or thyroid stimulating hormone (TSH) telling the thyroid gland to produce more T3 and T4. But again, having a pituitary gland that is functioning less than optimal will lead to some dysfunctional thyroid gland.

The moral: the organs and other tissues in the body inextricably connected therefore be cautious of being presented of "one size fits all" solution. So Keeping the thyroid gland healthy is making sure the rest of body is functioning normally and healthy.

Q7: What are the common tests for thyroid health issues?

A7: A good start to test the thyroid gland function is to check the TSH (thyroid stimulating hormone) if the TSH level is high that can indicate the thyroid gland is not functioning normally or in an optimal way and you can be diagnosed with hypothyroidism. And a low level of TSH that can indicate hyperthyroidism, however, a low TSH does not always mean a thyroid disorder but a pituitary gland problem and can be diagnosed with a secondary hypothyroidism.

Testing for Thyroxine (T4): there is a Free T4 and **bound-to-proteins T4,** and the focus is on FT4 where it can enter cells, not the other one. High FT4 is associated with hyperthyroidism, and low FT4 is associated with hypothyroidism. Having a blood test for FT4 and TSH together provides a more accurate diagnosis.

Triiodothyronine (T3): abnormally high levels of T3 and low TSH is more indicative and helpful for diagnosing patients with hyperthyroidism than hypothyroidism.

Test for Thyroid Antibodies: One of the antibodies to test for is the thyroid-stimulating immunoglobulins (TSI) to see if you have an autoimmune condition affecting the thyroid gland and indicating that you might have Graves' disease which leads to hyperthyroidism.

Another antibody to test for is called the Thyroid peroxidase (**TPO**) that can explain the presence of autoimmune disorder which is implicated with Hashimoto's or even Graves' disease.

CHAPTER SEVEN: Conclusion

The thyroid hormones (T4 and the T3) produced by the 2-inch thyroid gland play vital roles in regulating the metabolic processes responsible for the production of enough energy within the body.

Because of this metabolic importance, several body functions are attributable to a healthy thyroid: enhanced growth and development, alteration of the harmful cholesterol levels and breaking down of sugars and fat to produce energy among the many other health importance.

The positive contributions of the thyroid depend on certain factors. Understanding the relationship between the thyroid and the determinants is helpful in ensuring a balance within the thyroid for healthy living: the gluten-thyroid relationship, pregnancy and thyroid health, stress-thyroid relationship and the diet-thyroid relationship among the other factors explained earlier in this book (not limited to the above).

Any undesirable alteration of these associations leads to an imbalance of the thyroid hence overproduction (hyperthyroidism) or the underproduction (hypothyroidism) of thyroid hormones. These are the common thyroid disorders. The burden of these conditions is estimated to be extremely high with 20 million Americans suffering from the different thyroid malfunctions. Depending on the type of thyroid issue, there are different causes responsible. For example, the problem with the pituitary gland, genetic defects, autoimmune disorders, excess iodine, and thyroiditis. Individuals suffering from the various thyroid conditions experience certain undesirable effects that play a role in the diagnosis of the thyroid conditions.

The problem arises since most symptoms of thyroid conditions are non-specific and hence making it difficult for the diagnosis. Professional doctors, however, have come with primary strategy in containing the adverse thyroid conditions. They advocate for early diagnosis before the complications worsen. However, there are challenges that have resulted to frequent misdiagnosis and hence made it a difficult endeavor in the quest to reset our thyroid. For example, the use of outdated TSH ranges, incompetency of the health professionals and the inability of the general population to detect the symptoms of a disorder. The doctors request their clients, therefore, to conduct the thyroid hormone test regularly to confirm their thyroid health.

There are different treatment options for a reliable thyroid. A four-step Neuro-Metabolic Treatment plan provides key principles in the management of a disoriented thyroid: modified diet, modified lifestyle, the use of nutritional supplements and the Brain Based Therapy. With regard to this NMT plan, there are many treatment procedures specific for the different thyroid condition. For instance, the thyroid replacement therapy is only used for the management of hypothyroidism while thyroid surgery is specific to hyperthyroidism. Many people prefer the natural medications to the synthetic ones. However, the different treatment options have individualized components that favor different personalities. It is, therefore, important to use the treatment procedures under the supervision of a qualified health practitioner.

Many questions have arisen following the increased incidence and prevalence of the adverse thyroid gland. Responses to a selection of such concerns have been responded to with the aim of increasing awareness about the thyroid conditions and their effects on the general health.

It is the responsibility of both the health practitioners and his or her clients to ensure a thyroid condition-free globe. Let everyone embrace the need to protect our thyroid gland for maximum body productivity.

Finally, if you enjoyed this book, please take the time to share your thoughts and post a review on Amazon. It would be greatly appreciated! Thank you and good luck!

www.ingramcontent.com/pod-product-compliance
Lightning Source LLC
Chambersburg PA
CBHW061225180526
45170CB00003B/1159